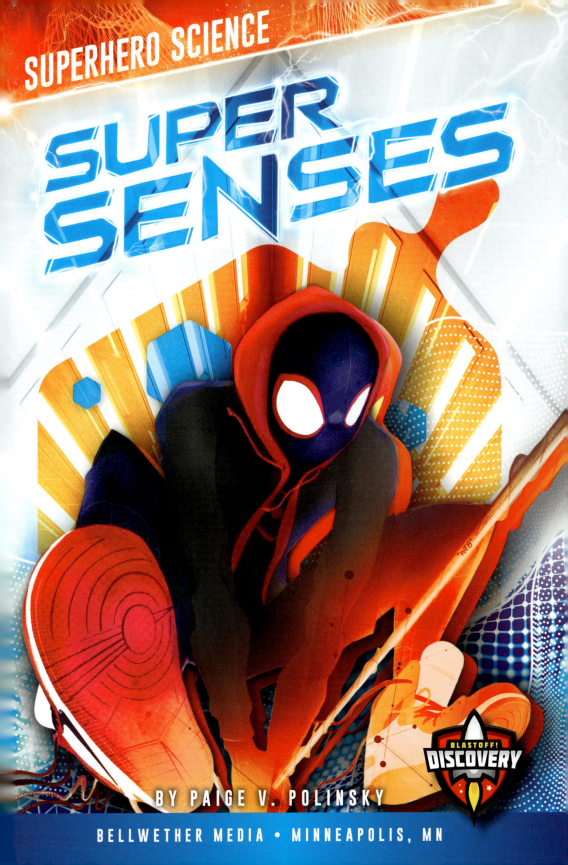

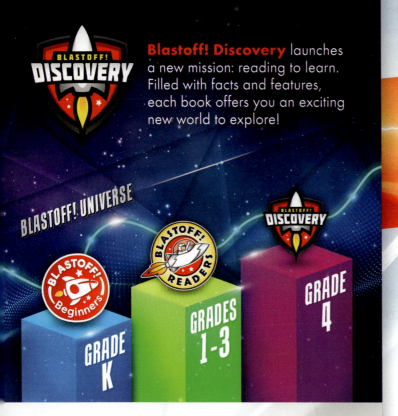

This edition first published in 2021 by Bellwether Media, Inc.

No part of this publication may be reproduced in whole or in part without written permission of the publisher.
For information regarding permission, write to Bellwether Media, Inc., Attention: Permissions Department,
6012 Blue Circle Drive, Minnetonka, MN 55343.

Library of Congress Cataloging-in-Publication Data

Names: Polinsky, Paige V., author.
Title: Super senses / by Paige V. Polinsky.
Description: Minneapolis, MN : Bellwether Media, 2021. |
Series: Blastoff! discovery : Superhero science | Includes bibliographical references and index. | Audience: Ages 7-13 | Audience: Grades 4-6 |
Summary: "Engaging images accompany information about the science of super senses. The combination of high-interest subject matter and narrative text is intended for students in grades 3 through 8"– Provided by publisher.
Identifiers: LCCN 2020017761 (print) | LCCN 2020017762 (ebook) | ISBN 9781644872611 (library binding) | ISBN 9781681037240 (ebook)
Subjects: LCSH: Senses and sensation–Juvenile literature. | Superheroes–Juvenile literature.
Classification: LCC QP434 .P64 2021 (print) | LCC QP434 (ebook) | DDC 612.8–dc23
LC record available at https://lccn.loc.gov/2020017761
LC ebook record available at https://lccn.loc.gov/2020017762

Text copyright © 2021 by Bellwether Media, Inc. BLASTOFF! DISCOVERY and associated logos are trademarks and/or registered trademarks of Bellwether Media, Inc.

Editor: Elizabeth Neuenfeldt   Designer: Jeffrey Kollock

Printed in the United States of America, North Mankato, MN.

TABLE OF CONTENTS

CLOSE CALL	4
THE POWER OF FIVE	8
SUPER SENSES IN EVERYDAY LIFE	14
THE BODY ELECTRIC	18
SENSING CHANGES	26
GLOSSARY	30
TO LEARN MORE	31
INDEX	32

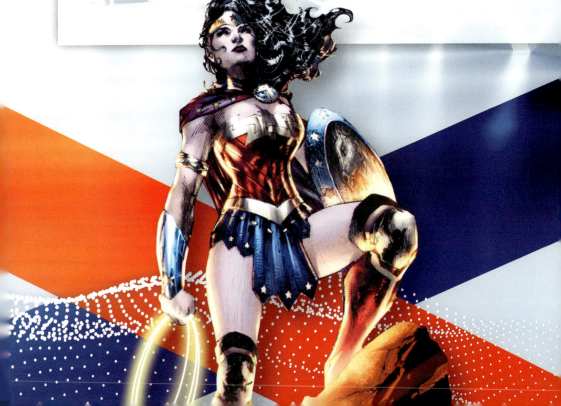

CLOSE CALL

Perched on a rooftop, Spider-Man looks over the city. He should be studying in his dorm. But his mentor's words echo in his head. With great power, there must also come great responsibility. Someone out there might need his help.

Suddenly, Spider-Man hears sirens. He looks below and notices two police cars speeding away in a flash of red and blue. Bingo. He leaps to his feet and dives off the edge of the building! Powerful threads fly from Spider-Man's wrist shooters. They stick to buildings like glue as he swings through the city.

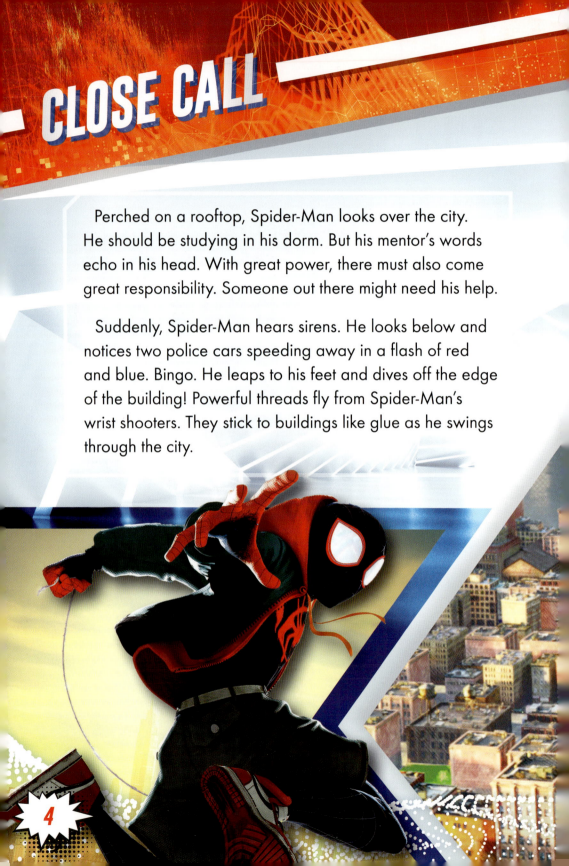

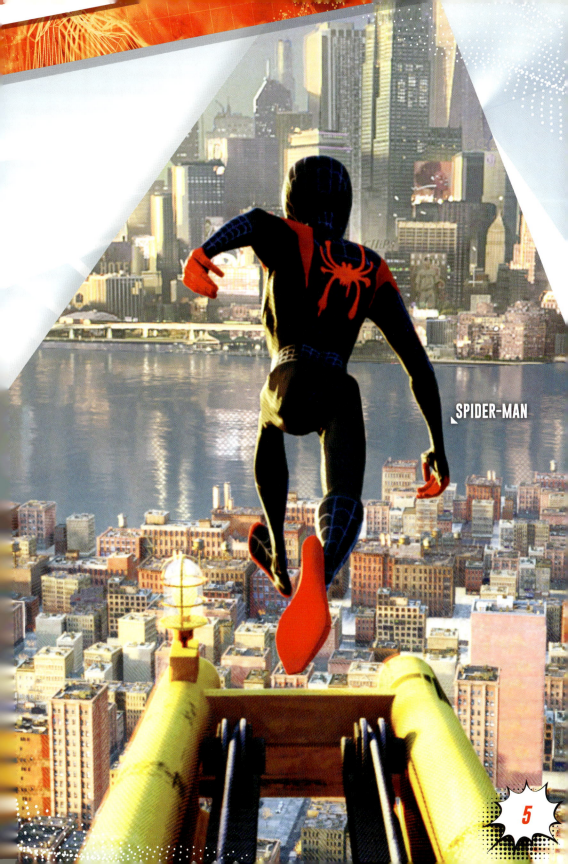

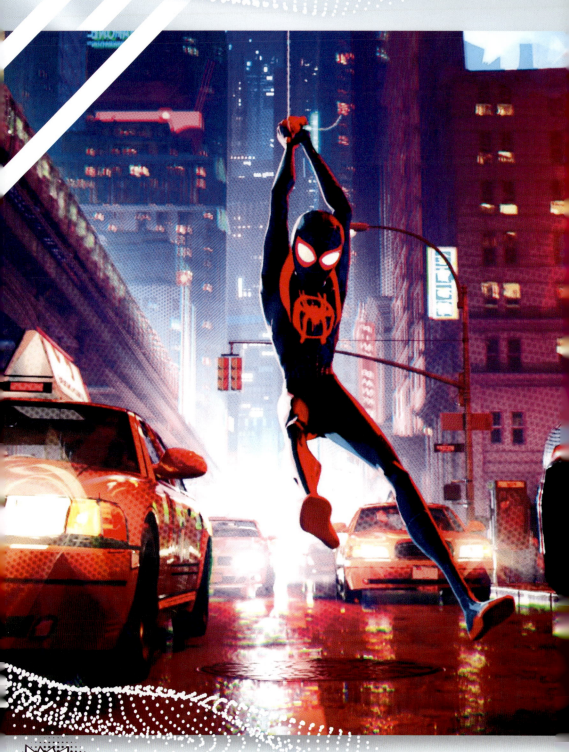

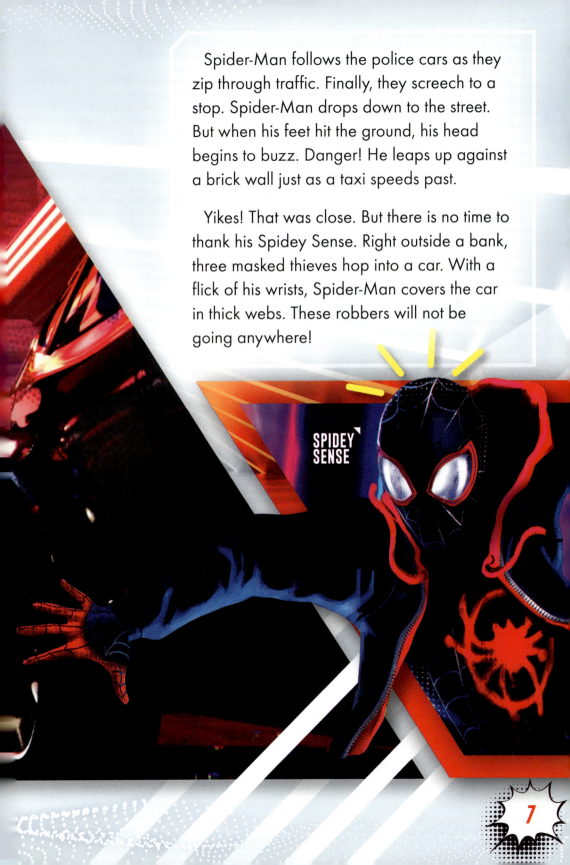

Spider-Man follows the police cars as they zip through traffic. Finally, they screech to a stop. Spider-Man drops down to the street. But when his feet hit the ground, his head begins to buzz. Danger! He leaps up against a brick wall just as a taxi speeds past.

Yikes! That was close. But there is no time to thank his Spidey Sense. Right outside a bank, three masked thieves hop into a car. With a flick of his wrists, Spider-Man covers the car in thick webs. These robbers will not be going anywhere!

THE POWER OF FIVE

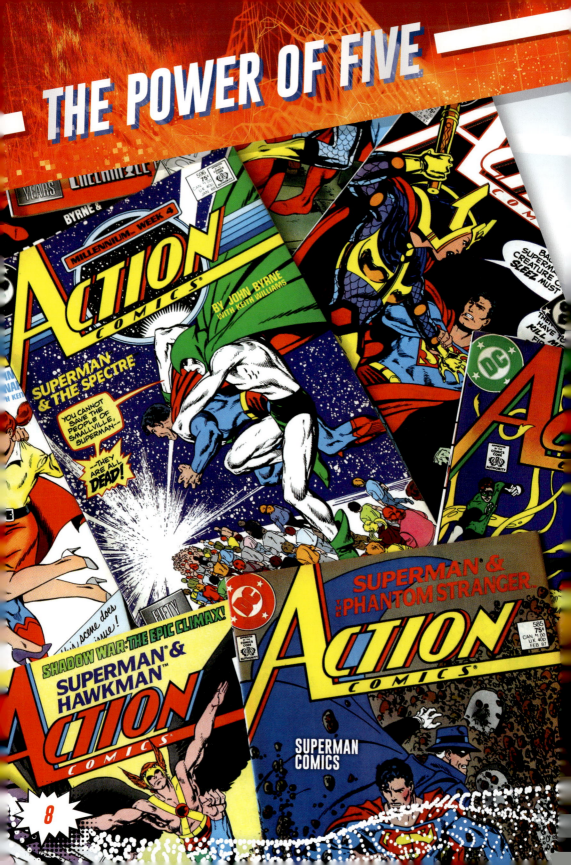

Our five senses help us explore the world. We can see new movies, listen to music, or feel cold on a chilly day. We also can smell and taste our favorite foods! In comics and movies, some of our favorite superheroes have super senses. They can sense things we cannot. They use super senses to save the day!

Many superheroes have **enhanced** vision. In 1938, DC Comics introduced Superman. He can see through walls! A few years later, Aquaman appeared alongside Superman. He can see thousands of feet below the water's surface!

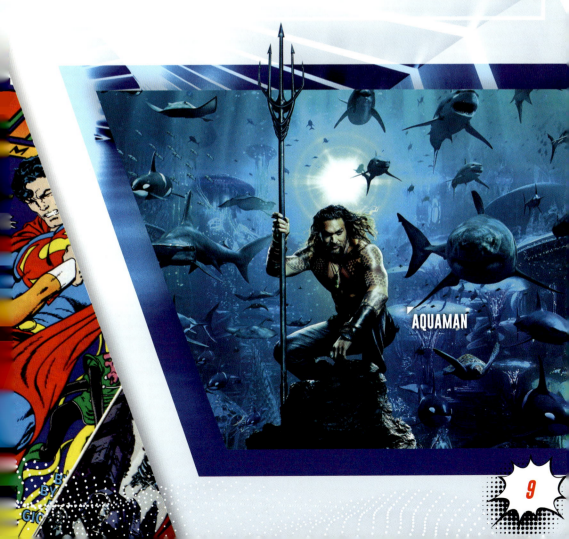

AQUAMAN

Some heroes have incredible hearing. In the 1940s, DC Comics introduced Wonder Woman. She was born with super hearing! Then in 1964, Marvel Comics created Daredevil. He is blind, but he uses his hearing and other super senses to sense and fight enemies. He can hear **ultrasonic** sounds. He can even tell if someone is lying by hearing their heartbeat!

Daredevil also has a great sense of taste. He can taste odors in the air. This helps him learn information about his surroundings!

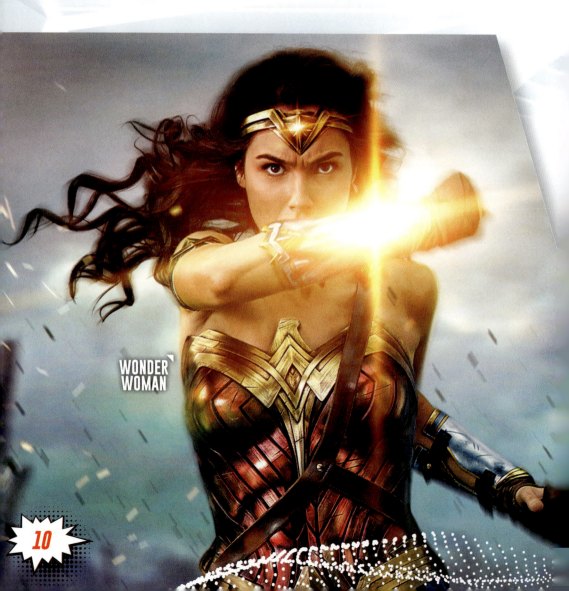
WONDER WOMAN

SUPERHERO PROFILE

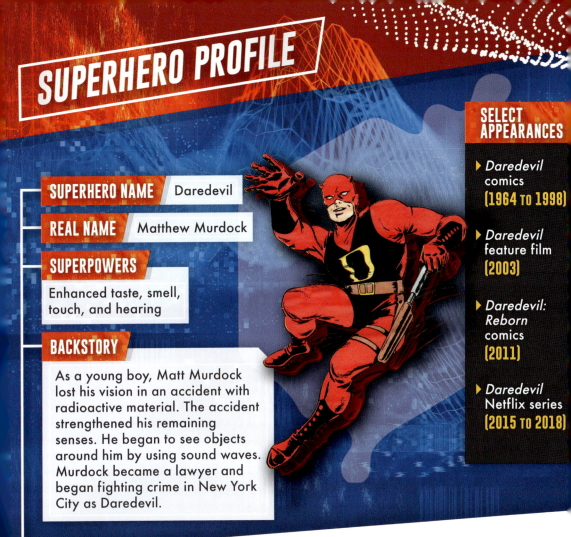

SUPERHERO NAME Daredevil

REAL NAME Matthew Murdock

SUPERPOWERS Enhanced taste, smell, touch, and hearing

BACKSTORY As a young boy, Matt Murdock lost his vision in an accident with radioactive material. The accident strengthened his remaining senses. He began to see objects around him by using sound waves. Murdock became a lawyer and began fighting crime in New York City as Daredevil.

SELECT APPEARANCES

- *Daredevil* comics (1964 to 1998)
- *Daredevil* feature film (2003)
- *Daredevil: Reborn* comics (2011)
- *Daredevil* Netflix series (2015 to 2018)

THE BLUE EAR

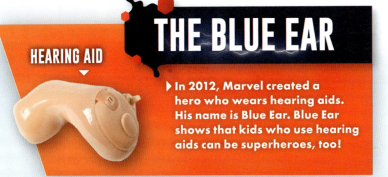

HEARING AID

▶ In 2012, Marvel created a hero who wears hearing aids. His name is Blue Ear. Blue Ear shows that kids who use hearing aids can be superheroes, too!

11

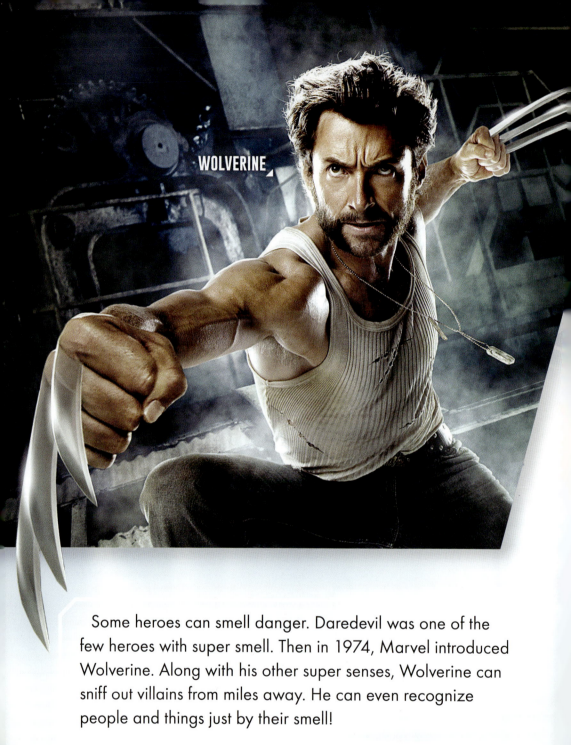

WOLVERINE

Some heroes can smell danger. Daredevil was one of the few heroes with super smell. Then in 1974, Marvel introduced Wolverine. Along with his other super senses, Wolverine can sniff out villains from miles away. He can even recognize people and things just by their smell!

Other heroes have enhanced touch. In the 1960s, Spider-Man was introduced with a Spidey Sense. He can sense danger before it even arrives! Since 1981, X-Men's Rogue has taken the power of touch even further. She can steal a person's memories, strength, and superpowers by touch alone!

MEDIA MANIA!

TV SERIES

Avatar: The Last Airbender

YEARS 2005 to 2008

DESCRIPTION

Many of the show's characters can control, or bend, different elements. Toph Beifong is a blind earthbender. She can feel the earth's vibrations to sense the world around her!

SUPER SENSES IN EVERYDAY LIFE

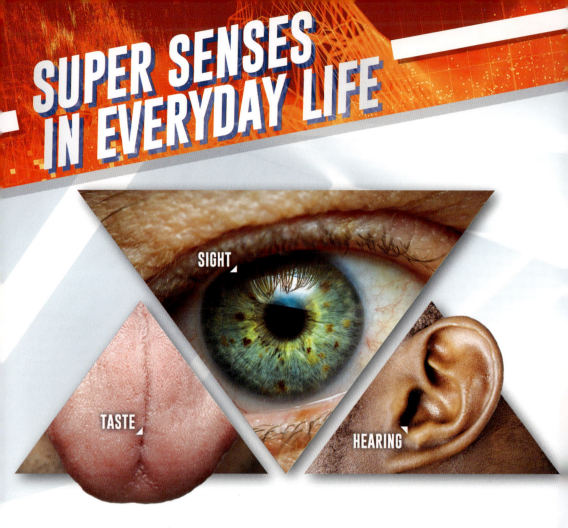

Some humans have natural super senses. The average person can see around one million colors. In rare cases, people are born with an extra **cone**. They can see 100 million colors! About one in four people are supertasters. Their extra **taste receptors** make flavors super intense!

The human brain can easily adapt, too. If one sense is damaged or lost, the brain works hard to make the other senses stronger. For example, a blind man named Daniel Kish uses his ears to see. He created a technique called flash sonar. Kish uses **echolocation** to "see" while riding his bike!

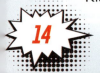

TASTE THE RAINBOW?

▶ A rare condition called synesthesia links different senses together. Some people with synesthesia see colors when they hear words. Others hear sounds that match flavors they taste. Many are amazing artists!

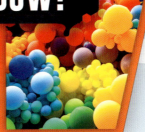

FLASH SONAR

1 A biker creates sound waves by clicking with their mouth.

2 Those sound waves travel and hit a tree.

3 Echoes bounce off the tree and return to the biker's ear, giving the biker a idea of the tree's size, shape, and location.

4 The biker successfully steers around the tree!

Everyday technologies can enhance our vision. **Microscopes** magnify images of very small things that the human eye cannot see. For example, scientists use them to learn more about **molecules**. People use **telescopes** to see things that are far away. Since the 1600s, they have helped people see stars that are millions of miles away!

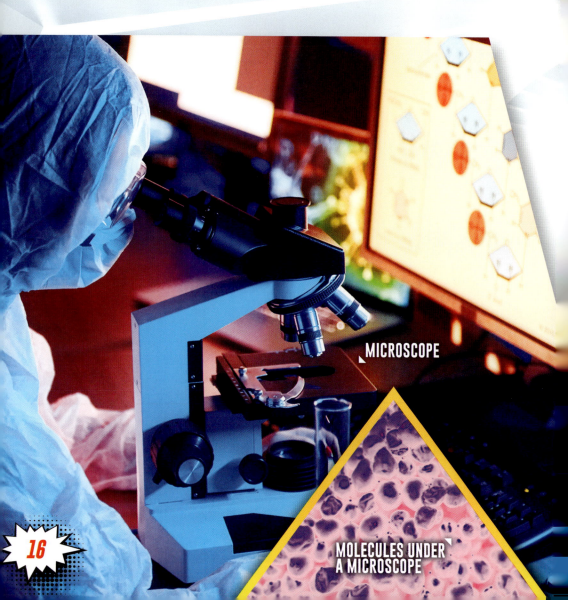

MICROSCOPE

MOLECULES UNDER A MICROSCOPE

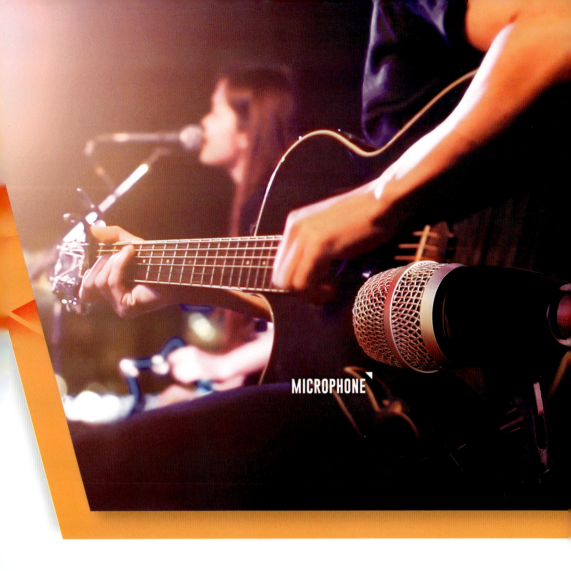

MICROPHONE

Other technologies help us hear better. **Microphones** and speakers work together to sense and **amplify** sounds. They help us listen to our favorite bands at noisy concerts, or talk with friends over the phone!

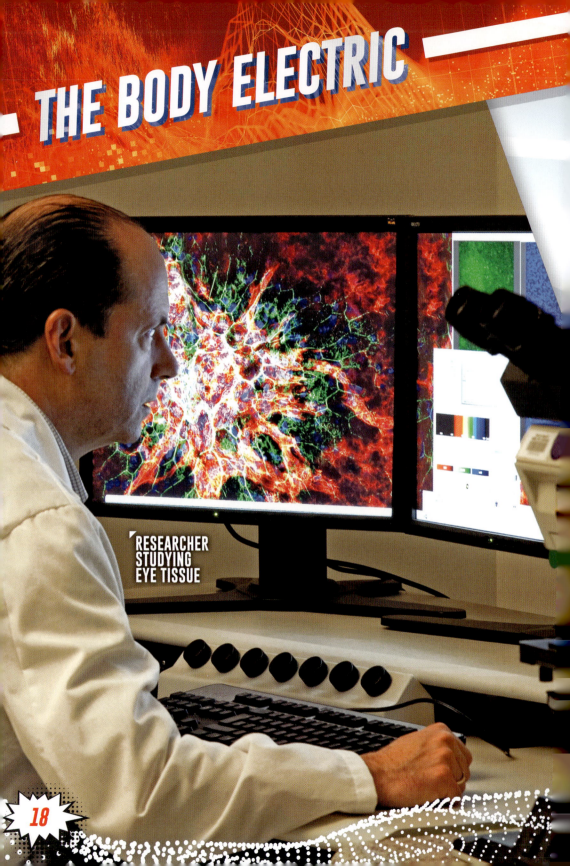

THE BODY ELECTRIC

RESEARCHER STUDYING EYE TISSUE

Right now, researchers are developing ways to restore lost or damaged senses. In 2019, researchers created robotic **contacts**. The lenses are fitted with **electrodes** that allow users to zoom in on something just by blinking twice! This could help people regain or even enhance their vision.

In the same year, Ocumetics began testing a new **bionic** lens. It is designed to replace a person's natural eye lens. It will take time before people can use them. But the device could restore eyesight at all distances!

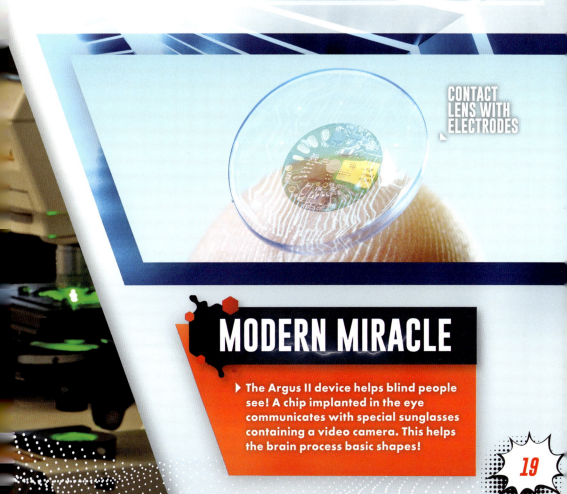

CONTACT LENS WITH ELECTRODES

MODERN MIRACLE

▶ The Argus II device helps blind people see! A chip implanted in the eye communicates with special sunglasses containing a video camera. This helps the brain process basic shapes!

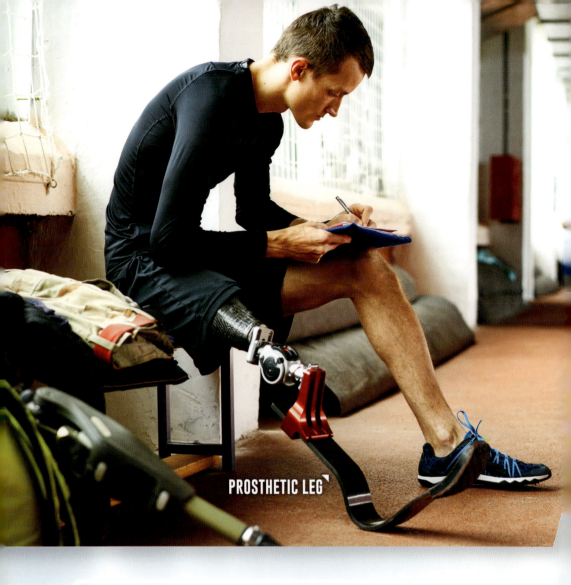

PROSTHETIC LEG

Scientists are also trying to help people regain a lost sense of touch. Up to 54 million people worldwide need **prostheses**. But prostheses can be hard to control because users have lost their sense of touch on their lost limb. In 2019, **engineers** made an electronic skin for prostheses that senses temperature and **pressure**!

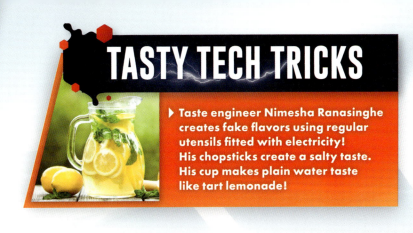

TASTY TECH TRICKS

▶ Taste engineer Nimesha Ranasinghe creates fake flavors using regular utensils fitted with electricity! His chopsticks create a salty taste. His cup makes plain water taste like tart lemonade!

Researchers are also fitting modern prosthetic devices with **sensors**. Electronic **signals** send information to the brain through wires. This allows users to feel pressure! However, prostheses are very expensive. Most people would not be able to afford these high-tech models.

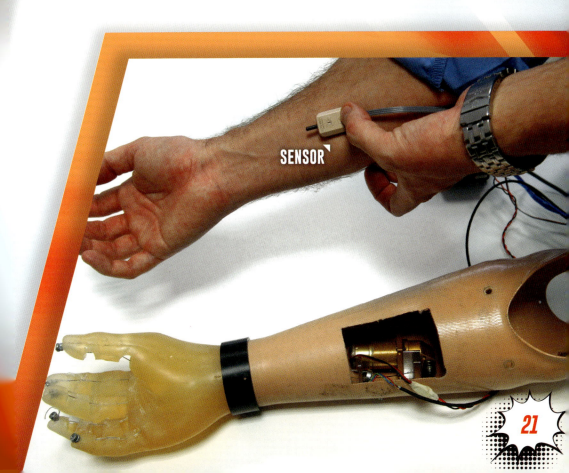

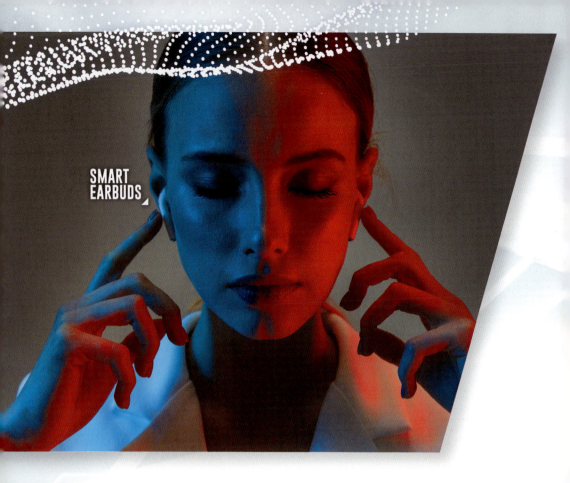

SMART EARBUDS

Some developers are creating tools to enhance senses. Doppler Lab's Here One earbuds could let users enhance specific sounds around them. But more research is needed before we could use them. They could enhance too many sounds by mistake and cause some to experience **sensory overload**.

To enhance touch, engineer Victor Mateevitsi made the SpiderSense suit in 2013. It allows wearers to sense objects within 60 feet (18 meters) around them. The suit contains tiny **mechanical** arms with ultrasonic microphones. When the microphones pick up sound, the arms apply a tingling pressure in the direction of the object.

THE NEGATIVE EFFECTS OF SUPER SENSES ON HUMANS

X-RAY VISION
EFFECTS:
- SENSORY OVERLOAD
- X-RAYS ARE VERY DANGEROUS AND COULD CAUSE CANCER

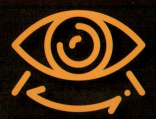

SUPER HEARING
EFFECTS:
- SENSORY OVERLOAD
- DIFFICULTY TUNING OUT BACKGROUND NOISE
- LOSS OF BALANCE

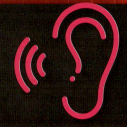

SUPER SMELL
EFFECTS:
- SENSORY OVERLOAD
- MIGRAINES
- ANXIETY

ENHANCED TOUCH
EFFECTS:
- SENSORY OVERLOAD
- LOWER PAIN THRESHOLD

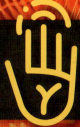

SUPER TASTE
EFFECTS:
- MALNUTRITION FROM PICKY EATING
- FREQUENT DROOLING
- MAY EAT NONFOOD ITEMS

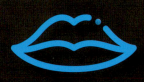

Other technology could give people super taste and smell. In 2019, IBM developed an electronic tongue! The device has sensors to detect salts, sugars, and other chemicals in liquids. The sensors are like robotic **taste buds**! Then the device processes that information to identify taste. This technology could help protect people with food allergies.

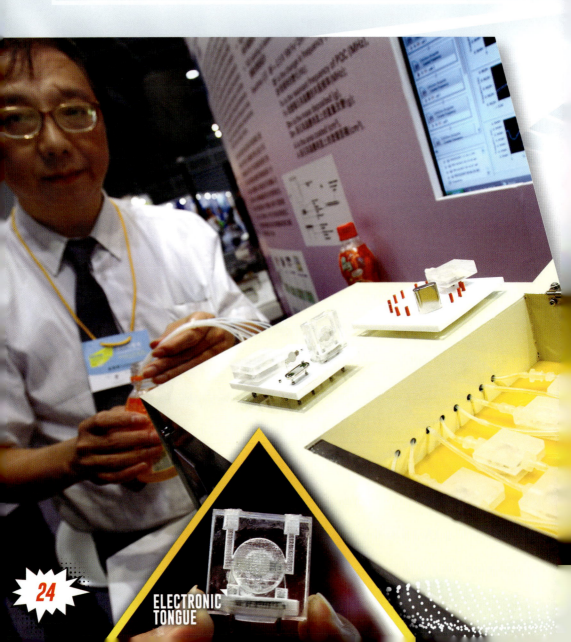

ELECTRONIC TONGUE

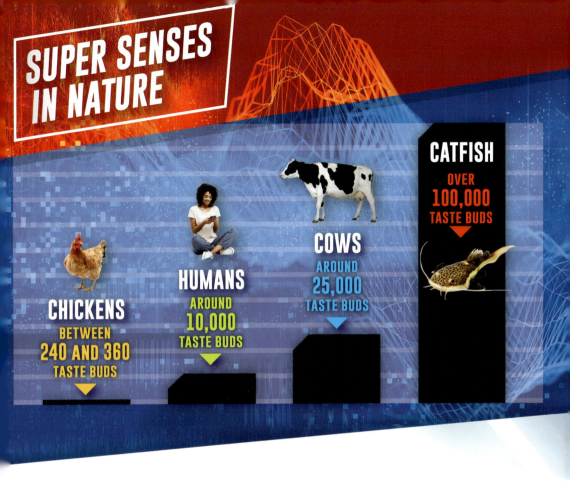

SUPER SENSES IN NATURE

CHICKENS BETWEEN 240 AND 360 TASTE BUDS

HUMANS AROUND 10,000 TASTE BUDS

COWS AROUND 25,000 TASTE BUDS

CATFISH OVER 100,000 TASTE BUDS

Scientists have developed several devices that smell out explosives. They could save many lives! Food companies are making mechanical noses to make sure their products are fresh. They can protect people from eating rotten food.

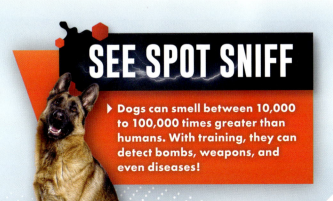

SEE SPOT SNIFF

▶ Dogs can smell between 10,000 to 100,000 times greater than humans. With training, they can detect bombs, weapons, and even diseases!

SENSING CHANGES

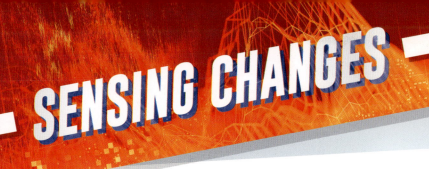

Human senses are complex. Scientists still have many questions about how they work. For now, much research is dedicated to restoring or improving damaged senses. Sight and hearing are top priorities.

Researchers are exploring taste and smell, too. Enhancing these senses could make us healthier! Some scientists are working to alter the human brain to enjoy vegetables more and sweets less. Hospitals could use similar technology to make food more enjoyable for recovering patients.

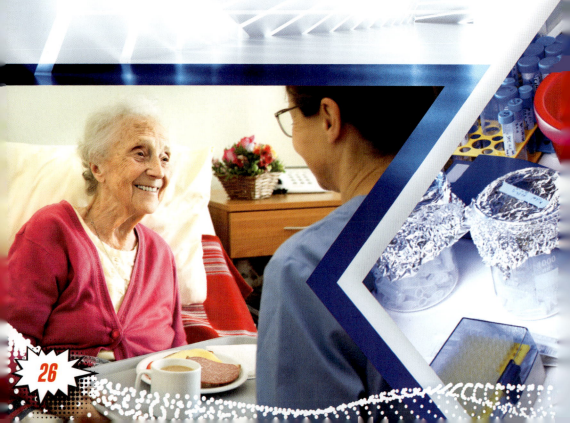

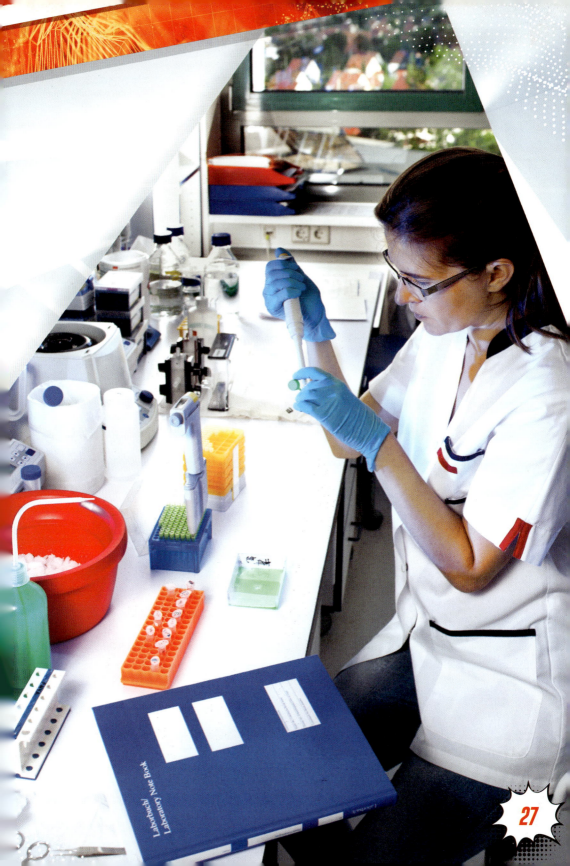

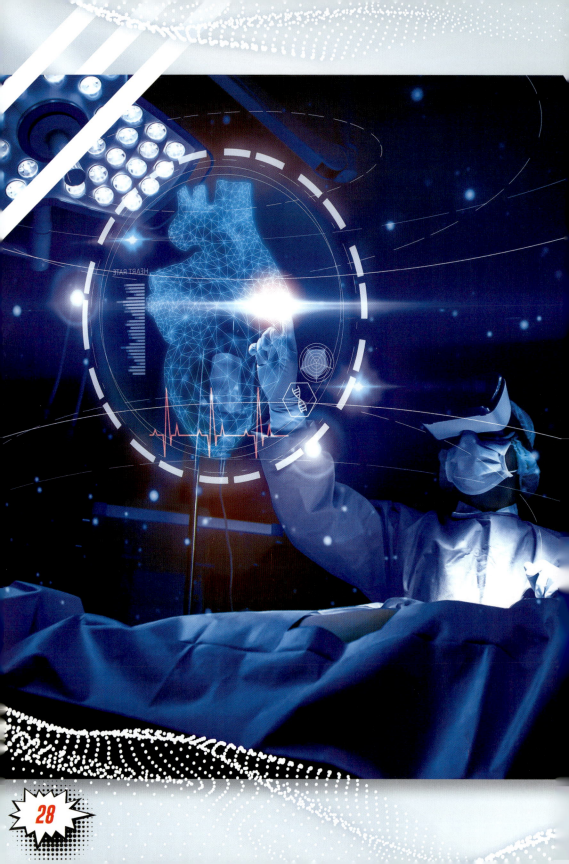

Using super sight, detectives could find the tiniest clues at crime scenes. Doctors with super senses could sniff out illnesses faster and more accurately. They could X-ray patients and check their heartbeats just by looking at them!

More and more tools are available to aid senses. In time, research may turn toward boosting human senses to superhuman levels. People may never have the same super senses as Superman or Wonder Woman. But future advances may lead to super senses that change how we explore our world!

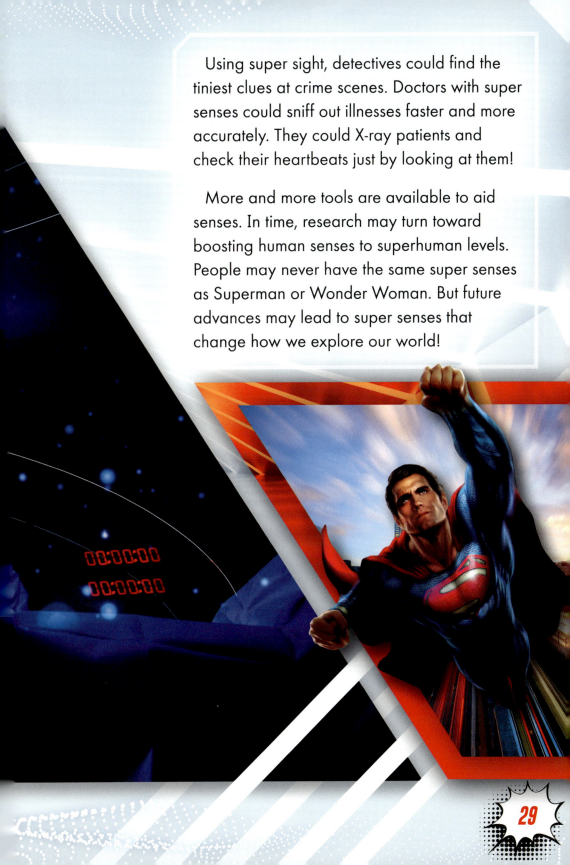

GLOSSARY

amplify—to make louder or greater

bionic—related to having body parts improved by technology

cone—a part of the eye that senses colored light

contacts—thin pieces of round plastic that are worn on the eyes to improve vision

echolocation—the process of locating objects by making sound waves and listening to the sound waves that are reflected back

electrodes—metallic points from which electricity can flow in or out

engineers—people who design and build machines

enhanced—made greater or better

mechanical—relating to something that is made or used by a machine

microphones—devices people use to record or amplify their voices

microscopes—devices that use lenses to help people see things that are very small by making them appear larger

molecules—the smallest parts of a substance having all the properties of the substance

pressure—the amount of power or force placed onto something

prostheses—man-made devices that replace or repair missing or injured parts of the body

sensors—devices that detect or sense heat, light, sound, or motion and react to it in a certain way

sensory overload—a condition in which a person gets more input from the five senses than the brain can process; sensory overload can cause discomfort, stress, headaches, sleeplessness, and dizziness.

signals—messages that serve to start some action

taste buds—groups of taste receptors that sense sweet, salty, sour, bitter, or savory things

taste receptors—the parts of taste buds that send messages about taste to the brain

telescopes—devices that have lenses to see objects that are far away

ultrasonic—relating to sounds that are too high for humans to hear

TO LEARN MORE

AT THE LIBRARY

Biskup, Agnieszka. *Seeing Through Walls: Superman and the Science of Sight.* North Mankato, Minn.: Capstone Press, 2016.

Duhig, Holly. *Bionic Limbs.* New York, N.Y.: Gareth Stevens Publishing, 2018.

Scirri, Kaitlin. *The Science of Invisibility and X-Ray Vision.* New York, N.Y.: Cavendish Square, 2019.

ON THE WEB

FACTSURFER

Factsurfer.com gives you a safe, fun way to find more information.

1. Go to www.factsurfer.com.

2. Enter "super senses" into the search box and click 🔍.

3. Select your book cover to see a list of related content.

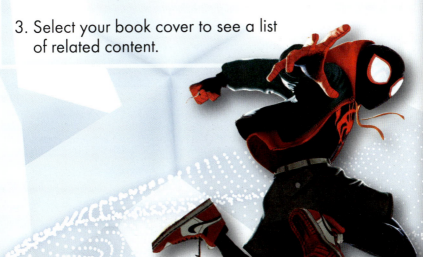

INDEX

Aquaman, 9
Argus II, 19
Avatar: The Last Airbender, 13
bionic lens, 19
Blue Ear, 11
cone, 14
contacts, 19
Daredevil, 10, 11, 12
DC Comics, 9, 10
echolocation, 14
effects on humans, 22, 23
electrodes, 19
electronic tongue, 24
flash sonar, 14, 15
hearing, 9, 10, 11, 14, 15, 17, 22, 23, 26
Here One, 22
Kish, Daniel, 14
Marvel Comics, 10, 11, 12
mechanical noses, 25
microphones, 17, 22
microscopes, 16
molecules, 16
prostheses, 20, 21
Rogue, 13

sensors, 21, 24
sensory overload, 22
smell, 9, 12, 23, 24, 25, 26, 29
Spider-Man, 4, 5, 7, 13
SpiderSense suit, 22
Spidey Sense, 7, 13
super senses in nature, 25
Superman, 8, 9, 29
synesthesia, 15
taste, 9, 10, 14, 15, 21, 23, 24, 25, 26
taste buds, 24, 25
taste receptors, 14
telescopes, 16
touch, 9, 13, 20, 21, 22, 23
vision, 9, 14, 15, 16, 19, 23, 26, 29
Wolverine, 12
Wonder Woman, 10, 29
X-Men, 13

The images in this book are reproduced through the courtesy of: AF archive/ Alamy, front cover (Spider-Man), p. 7 (Spidey Sense); Creative Stock/ Alamy, p. 3 (Wonder Woman); Columbia Pictures/ Courtesy Everett Collection, pp. 4, 4-5, 31; Album/ Alamy, pp. 6-7, 29 (Superman); Art Directors & TRIP/ Alamy, pp. 8-9 (Superman comics); PictureLux/ The Hollywood Archive/ Alamy, p. 9 (Aquaman); Art Villone/ Alamy, p. 11 (Daredevil); Jiri Hera, p. 11 (hearing aid); Photo 12/ Alamy, pp. 12-13 (Wolverine); Wiki Commons, p. 13 (PixieMe, p. 14 (taste); Nik Bruining, p. 14 (sight); B-D-S Piotr Marcinski, p. 14 (sound); lazyllama, p. 15 (synesthesia); Ljupco Smokovski, p. 15 (step 1, 3, biker), (step 4 biker); kpboonjit, p. 15 (step 2, 3, 4 biker); Standret, pp. 16-17 (microscope); Panther Media GmbH/ Alamy, p. 16 (molecules); PopTika, pp. 16-17 (microphone); BSIP SA/ Alamy pp. 18-19 (researcher); HQuality, p. 19 (contact lens); SeventyFour pp. 20-21 (prosthetic leg); Oksana Shufrych, p. 21 (lemonade); Dino Fracchia/ Alamy, p. 21 (sensor); Dean Drobot, pp. 22 (smart earbuds), 25 (human); South China Morning Post/ Contributor/ Getty Images, pp. 24-25, 24 (electronic tongue); Olhastock, p. 25 (chicken); Eric Isselee, p. 25 (cow); livingpitty, p. 25 (catfish); gualtiero boffi, p. 25 (dog); FredFroese, p. 26; anyaivanova, pp. 26-27; Fit Ztudio, pp. 28-29.